Healthy BEGINNINGS

A Holistic Approach to Preconception, Pregnancy, and Parenting

Dr. Felicity Keough-Bligh

Healthy Beginnings

A Holistic Approach to Preconception, Pregnancy, and Parenting

Dr. Felicity Keough-Bligh

Published by Three Peas Press, St. Charles, MO

Copyright ©2024 Dr. Felicity Keough-Bligh

All rights reserved.

No part of this publication may be reproduced, stored in a retrieval system, or transmitted in any form or by any means, electronic, mechanical, photocopying, recording, scanning, or otherwise, except as permitted under Section 107 or 108 of the 1976 United States Copyright Act, without the prior written permission of the Publisher. Requests to the Publisher for permission should be addressed to the Permissions Department, Three Peas Press, dr.keough@keoughchiropractic.com.

Limit of Liability/Disclaimer of Warranty: While the publisher and author have used their best efforts in preparing this book, they make no representations or warranties with respect to the accuracy or completeness of the contents of this book and specifically disclaim any implied warranties of merchantability or fitness for a particular purpose. No warranty may be created or extended by sales representatives or written sales materials. The advice and strategies contained herein may not be suitable for your situation. You should consult with a professional where appropriate. Neither the publisher nor the author shall be liable for any loss of profit or any other commercial damages, including but not limited to special, incidental, consequential, or other damages.

The product information and advice provided (in this book) are intended for general informational purposes only. The author and publisher of this book have made every effort to ensure that the content is accurate and up to date at the time of publication. However, they make no representations or warranties of any kind, express or implied, about the completeness, accuracy, reliability, suitability, or availability of the information, products, or services contained in this book for any purpose.

Project Management and Book Design: Davis Creative, LLC, dba: Davis CreativePublishing.com

Publisher's Cataloging-in-Publication

Names: Keough-Bligh, Felicity, author.

Title: Healthy beginnings : a holistic approach to preconception, pregnancy, and parenting / Dr. Felicity Keough-Bligh.

Description: St. Charles, MO : Three Peas Press, [2024]

Identifiers: ISBN: 978-1-7341840-4-4 (paperback) | 978-1-7341840-3-7 (ebook) | LCCN: 2024916517

Subjects: LCSH: Pregnancy--Health aspects. | Chiropractic. | Preconception care. | Postnatal care. | Parenting--Health aspects. | BISAC: MEDICAL / Nursing / Maternity, Perinatal, Women's Health. | MEDICAL / Nursing / Pediatric & Neonatal. | MEDICAL / Chiropractic.

Classification: LCC: RG525 .K46 2024 | DDC: 618.2--dc23

ATTENTION CORPORATIONS, UNIVERSITIES, COLLEGES, AND PROFESSIONAL ORGANIZATIONS: Quantity discounts are available on bulk purchases of this book for educational, gift purposes, or as premiums for increasing magazine subscriptions or renewals. Special books or book excerpts can also be created to fit specific needs. For information, please contact Three Peas Press, dr.keough@keoughchiropractic.com.

*To my husband Luke
and my children
Preston Joseph and Parker Lee.
You are the loves of my life.*

ACKNOWLEDGMENTS

Plenty of people helped bring this book to fruition, and I am grateful to all of them.

First, I would like to thank my amazing husband, Luke. For always believing in me and supporting my dreams. For also keeping our little ones occupied so I could write. You were an important part of birthing this book.

I want to thank my sons for being my greatest teachers.

Thanks to everyone on the Davis Creative Publishing team who helped me so much. Special thanks to Cathy, Jack, Cheryl, and Julie. Thank you for believing in this work and helping me bring it into the world.

Thank you to all my patients for allowing me to be your friend and doctor and teaching me so much about health and healing over the years.

To my team members and colleagues at Keough Chiropractic, thank you for your shared passion for healing our community.

To my parents and sisters, Geoffrey, Susan, Mercedes, Tess, and Stephanie, for your encouragement and love.

To the reader, I want to recognize and acknowledge you for taking your health into your own hands.

Finally, I thank God for answering my prayers, making me an instrument of healing, and guiding my life all along the way.

TABLE OF CONTENTS

Introduction: What Our World Needs Now	1
The Three T's: Trauma, Toxins, And Thoughts	4
What Is Functional Medicine?	23
Preconception: Preparing for Baby	33
Pregnancy And Chiropractic	56
Pregnancy, Labor And Delivery with Chiropractic	57
How Can Chiropractic Care Help Me DurIng My Pregnancy, Labor, and Delivery?	60
Chiropractic Benefits for the Pregnant Women	62
Chiropractic Effects During Labor	65
What Do I Look for in a Chiropractor If I'm pregnant?	67
Should I Have a Chiropractor on My Birth Team?	69
What is the Webster Technique and How Does it Help Me Achieve a More Balanced Body and Baby?	71
Can Chiropractic Care Lessen Chances of Intervention At Birth?	73
Is Chiropractic During Pregnancy Safe?	76
Five Reasons Why Chiropractic Treatment Is Beneficial During Pregnancy	77
And Beyond…: Infants And Pediatric Chiropractic	81
Reasons For Your Child to be Checked by a Chiropractor	86
Next Steps	87
Biography	89
Endnotes	91

INTRODUCTION

WHAT OUR WORLD NEEDS NOW

Big decisions lie ahead. With so much turmoil and chaos in the world, it can be scary to think about bringing additional children into the world. Many adults talk to me about wanting to have children, but they are hesitant, and yes, there are many reasons to be cautious: current world affairs, the emotional and financial drain of dealing with prior infertility, a traumatic birth(s), sensory, spectrum or behavioral challenges in a child…the list goes on. While considering whether or not to have children, adults may not realize that healthy children are precisely what our world needs and each child needs parents who are being their best and healthiest selves. We have incredible research, validated information, and tried-and-tested resources available as never before to help make that big decision. We see it as an incredible opportunity to turn the tide for a healthier next generation and generations to come.

This book presents important aspects of *chiropractic: preconception, pregnancy, and beyond.* It covers broader information about how to live a life of greatness and pass it along to our children by creating greater adaptability and nourishing our health.

We've learned through the science of genetics and epigenetics[i] that we can literally change our genetic makeup depending on internal and external environmental factors, first and foremost the health of the nervous system, as well as diet and lifestyle.

My goal with this book and in my practice is to empower parents so they can change their epigenetics, beginning now before conception and through pregnancy and parenting so they may endure through future generations.

This book is a tool to help you decide and learn how to balance your nervous system, change your lifestyle, clean up your diet and environment, fix your gut and microbiome,[ii] and deal with emotional stressors. If you do this, you will have dramatic health changes you never thought possible.

I'd like to emphasize the importance of working with a neurologically trained chiropractor ***first.*** Before attempting to tackle everything at once, ensuring that your nervous system is balanced and the Vagus nerve is working properly, all other modalities we utilize to create health will be more effective.

This first chapter in this book covers the Three T's: Trauma, Toxins, and Thoughts, and provides alternative approaches to addressing the effects of stress, chemicals, and emotions in our children. The Three T's are urgent, escalating conditions that demand recognition and attention.

With this book, you will discover that you do not need to feel you are a victim of your "genetics." Science is now understanding that our genes change the way they "express" themselves based on our environment.

Finally, this book will ask and answer important questions about chiropractic care from preconception, to post delivery, and beyond. It includes an overview of Functional Medicine to help you compare and reflect on the importance of finding the right solutions to help you and your child or children attain a healthy body, mind, and interrelated, interconnected systems.

In health,

Dr. Felicity Keough-Bligh

THE THREE T'S:

TRAUMA, TOXINS, AND THOUGHTS

Because the beginning of a book is critically important for engaging the reader, I have chosen to make the first chapter about three things that are of great significance: The Three T's—Trauma (physical), Toxins (chemicals), and Thoughts (emotional). Before we dive into the first T and explore physical, neurological trauma, it is relevant to mention that trauma is the most overlooked of the three T's. Birth itself is a trauma. Many, if not most, babies are born undergoing a certain degree of trauma which will lay the groundwork for the health of the child in his/her lifetime. While Toxins (chemicals) and Thoughts (emotions) are a large part of the issue, long before the pandemic of 2020, birth trauma had been getting worse for decades. Over just two generations, rates of chronic illness in kids have risen to troubling levels.

- ADHD and Behavioral Problems in kids range from 10-15%, with rates continuing to climb.

- Anxiety in kids was 11.6%, then nearly doubled to 20.5% during the pandemic.

- Depression in kids was 8.5%, then more than doubled to 25.5% due to the pandemic.

- Overall, mental illness now affects 1 in 6 kids and is only increasing.
- Autism rates have increased 241% just since 2000, and now affects 1 in 44 kids.[iii]

Ten to twenty years is not enough time for genetics to change much. I've been fascinated with the study of genetics and epigenetics long before I went to college and studied them extensively. It was apparent to me that there was more to these chronic childhood health conditions than just *bad genes*, so I started looking deeper. Working with parents to assess their children's health history, I learned they were told that the reasons their children were struggling were the result of genetics or just bad luck. My intention isn't to downplay modern, Western medicine in this book but to shed light on the fact that not all the answers are genetic, and wrong answers will not help stop this growing issue in our children.

First T: Trauma

Trauma that results from birth intervention is not talked about in traditional medicine and mainstream health care; however, it is the missing link to the reason our children are chronically sick, with difficulty nursing, colic, reflux, constipation, ear infections, RSV infection, croup, chronic colds, allergies, asthma, and chronic autoimmune issues. It is also the missing link as to why children are chronically stressed, presenting with autism, sensory processing disorder,

ADHD, anxiety, depression, focus and learning challenges, and sleep disorders.

To ensure we have the healthiest children possible, the most important thing to do is educate ourselves and learn all we can to reduce The Three T's (trauma, toxins, thoughts) as much as possible to allow the full potential of the child's nervous system to develop. For children who are chronically sick and suffering, nothing matters more than figuring out exactly what caused them to get sick and struggle in the first place. After fifteen years of caring for thousands of babies and children, and working with everything from colic, nursing issues, constipation, chronic ear infections, sensory processing disorder, cerebral palsy, autism, and epilepsy, I can tell you with certainty there is one thing that stands out in most of those case histories that only a select few practitioners are talking about: the neurological birth trauma that happens to babies.

Above all else, we must address why the nervous system is out of balance due to things like induction, manual assistance, forceps, vacuum, and c-section, plus prenatal and maternal stress during pregnancy. This is not a new thing, but once 2020 hit, an enormous amount of additional stress was added to expecting mothers, making this situation worse.

Birth, Trauma, and the Brainstem

The bones of the skull, upper neck, and entire spine are so much more important than most realize. They give structure to the entire frame of the body, and they also house and protect the most important organ in our body–the central and autonomic nervous system. If these areas are physically injured or altered due to the birth process, the function of the body is also altered from the first moment of life and beyond. Vital functions of the nervous system include:

- Balance nerves and muscles responsible for digestion
- Balance nerves and muscles responsible for breastfeeding
- Balance nerves and muscles responsible for the drainage of fluid from ears and sinuses
- Balance all sensory processing: eyes, auditory, smell, touch
- Controls and regulates our motor development, milestones, balance, tone, coordination
- Balance and control speech function and development
- Balance the function of our immune system and inflammation.
- Controls and regulates ALL initial brain communication and coordination- social, emotional, behavioral, memory, and decision-making.

The nervous system controls every function in the body, but there is one key nerve that connects all the vital functions together: the Vagus Nerve. This very important nerve is what controls your baby's ability to open its mouth to latch, nurse, and digest breastmilk. It also controls the function of the immune system. When this nerve is working properly, babies are having bowel movements after feedings and are healthy and happy. When it is not working well, babies are constipated and sick. This nerve controls your child's neuromuscular system and motor development. It also is responsible for your child's ability to calm down and relax, listen to instructions, transition and to be able to fall (and stay) asleep at night. Lastly, it regulates our emotions and social interactions. The Vagus nerve is the number one vital nerve to your child's health and well-being.

Unfortunately, there are many factors in today's world that influence the Vagus nerve in a negative way:

- Maternal and prenatal stress and anxiety.

- Intervention and trauma during labor and delivery (forceps, vacuum extraction, c-section)

- Inflammatory foods and chemicals in our environment

- Childhood traumas (falls, bumps to head)

- Stress and anxiety in the family and in society.

Each of these can overwhelm or interfere with the Vagus Nerve and its ability to perform its functions, which are mostly rest, digestion, and healing. These stressors show up early and often in our children's lives and most of us don't even know it is happening. Once the brainstem area is altered or injured from birth, it initiates a condition that explains so many struggles that children face, called dysautonomia.

Oftentimes, when our children suffer, our pediatrician or family doctors tell us "Its normal, don't worry about it." Or "They will grow out of it." Children with reflux, colic, constipation, chronic colds, ear infections, and respiratory infections do not grow out of these issues; unfortunately, they grow into them, meaning they develop deeper and more chronic health issues.

- Babies with colic and constipation can grow into chronic ear and respiratory infections and are prescribed multiple rounds of antibiotics.

- Children with constant ear and respiratory infections can grow into chronic asthma and allergies.

- Children with chronic digestive and immune challenges early on can grow into speech, sensory, emotion and behavioral challenges.

- Children with hyperactivity can grow into stressed out, anxious, depressed teenagers.

Before we know it, our children become what we are: overwhelmed, exhausted, emotional adults. Many of us have been dealing with this layered stress upon stress since we were born. I believe that is why you are reading this book now, so you can learn there is hope and healing when we get the Vagus Nerve back to functioning as it was designed and balance the Nervous System through neurologically focused chiropractic care.

Sickness, Medications and Stress

As you review the following six stages of life, ask yourself if they were part of your experience or any previous parenting experience. These events often go from birth through adulthood:

1. Babies present fussy, gassy, colicky, and have sleep challenges

2. Challenging baby to toddler stage with sensory issues, constantly sick, repeatedly needing antibiotics and steroid-based anti-inflammatory medications.

3. Child is constantly wound up, hyperactive, impulsive, emotional, and sensory overwhelmed.

4. Older child is challenged in grade school and has trouble with concentration and focus, organization, social and emotional regulation.

5. Teenager struggles with anger, anxiety and depression.

6. Stressed out, overwhelmed, exhausted adult.

Many parents agree that this explains their child or even themselves growing up. The good news is more families than ever before are doing their own research and learning to be the best advocate for their children, as well as for themselves. Parents are turning to medications as a last resort and first choosing more natural ways to support their children. This is a very positive shift from a decade ago when many of the children I worked with in practice were on at least one-two psychotropic drugs that had many terrible side effects. I can say without a doubt that parents and families are making huge steps in the right direction for the health of their families.

Subluxation and Pediatric Chiropractic

All that we've discussed up to this point touched on the health issues that plague us and our children and the sequence of how the 3-T's impact our health. You are probably wondering at this point how are we going to get you the help you need. The answer is found in something you may have never considered: a neurologically focused and trained chiropractor, starting with Subluxation.

Subluxation

Subluxation is an important condition that is responsible for many sick children today. A subluxation consists of three main components:

1. Misalignment

2. Tension and Fixation

3. Neurological Interference and Imbalance

Subluxation can happen in any joint in the body, from your toes to your shoulders, but it is the subluxation of the spine and central nervous system that is the culprit of so much dysfunction and chronic illness in our children today.

What Causes Subluxation?

Stress and toxicity are the primary causes of subluxation. Normally, stress is part of a healthy life. Stress helps us gain strength, resiliency, and adaptability from the moment we come into this life. However, based on our observation and study of children's health, there is too much stress and toxicity in our current environment. The amount of stress and anxiety pregnant mothers face is more than ever before. Our hospital's labor and delivery rooms have turned birth into a medical event, instead of allowing the natural process of birth to unfold and only intervene when the health of the mother and child is in danger. Furthermore, every time a child is prescribed antibiotics under the age of three, it greatly increases their risk of chronic illness later in life.

Back to the Three T's: Traumas (physical), Toxins (chemicals), and Thoughts (emotional). Everyone faces these Three T's in life, but when our children face so many of them at such an early age, it allows Subluxation to set into the nervous system. Subluxation creates chronic and significant imbalance and dysfunction to the nervous system. When this happens, dysfunction is spread downstream to all other major systems: digestive, immune, respiratory, mental, and emotional.

Signs of Subluxation

Subluxation negatively affects the central nervous system, which is responsible for all our physiology and functions, because of this, subluxation can show up as many different signs and symptoms:

- Reflux
- Colic
- Nursing difficulties
- Sleeping challenges
- Digestive challenges
- Frequent emotional meltdowns and tantrums

- Focus and concentration issues
- Hyperactivity and impulsivity
- Emotional regulation challenges
- Chronic pain and tension
- Fatigue and exhaustion
- Movement disorders

How to Detect and Fix Subluxation

In our practice, our primary modes of finding subluxation include postural, physical, and neurological exam components. We also use radiographic imaging in specific cases, but the most important tool is called the INSIGHT Subluxation Scanning Technology. These scans find, measure, and locate dysautonomia (malfunction of the autonomic nervous system (ANS). The ANS is the part of the nervous system that controls involuntary bodily functions, such as heart rate, blood pressure, digestion, endocrine system, temperature regulation, and more) as well as other aspects of subluxation. Using this technology allows the creation of an exact, personalized, and customized plan of adjusting a child, teenager or adult.

Correction of the issue is simple yet powerful and complex at the same time. A trained pediatric and neurologically focused chiropractor is someone who uses an adjusting system that is safe, gentle, and extremely effective at restoring function and balance to the nervous system.

One of the most wonderful things about adjusting in this way is it doesn't take much time; it fits easily into the family's busy schedule and is also fun and enjoyable for the child!

To summarize, the nervous system is the absolute most important system of the body that regulates and controls every other major system in the body. The main control center is in the brainstem, which, as we discussed, is easily injured and damaged during the birth process for millions of children. When subluxation takes hold in the upper spine, it can remain stuck unless examined and treated by a pediatric chiropractor. Subluxation that presents from the birth process (and sometimes even before birth with malpositions such as breech, transverse presentations, or other prenatal challenges) will alter the most important of all infant and childhood brain development, movement, and motor milestones. These are intricately connected; without them, an entire host of previously discussed signs and symptoms will ensue. When subluxation is present, even in a mild form, dysautonomia will also present.

The Second T: Toxins

In this section, we will be discussing the second T: Toxins (chemicals) and how the chemicals in our environment before birth impact the health of our children.

Children are especially vulnerable to environmental threats due to their developing organs and immune systems, smaller bodies and airways. Harmful exposures can begin as early as in utero. Furthermore, breastfeeding can be a significant source of exposure to certain chemicals in infants; this should, however, not discourage breastfeeding, which carries numerous positive health and developmental benefits that far outweigh commercial formula. In some instances, when the mother cannot breastfeed her baby, using a homemade formula that closely mimics the breastmilk component is recommended over commercial formulas. Proportionate to the child's size, children ingest more food, drink more water, and breathe more air than adults. Additionally, certain modes of behavior, such as putting hands and objects into the mouth and playing outdoors can increase children's exposure to environmental contaminants. In short, we live in a world that can be extremely toxic to our health, whether we are unborn children or more than one hundred years old, and our bodies are constantly being burdened by chemicals and attempting to mitigate the effects on our health.

Despite our constant toxic exposure, it is important to understand that more parents than ever before are choosing to educate themselves on ways to reduce toxin exposure in their homes. We may not be able to control what we breathe and eat when we walk outside our home, but more and more families are intentionally looking for ways to clean up their home environments, including:

- Nontoxic cleaning and cooking products
- Organic, gluten-free, casein-free, dye-free foods
- Using essential oils in place of toxic scents and air fresheners

Each of these and other changes in the home environment helps reduce the family's toxic exposure. Parents are also opting for medication as a last resort (due to side effects) and choosing high-quality nutrition, supplements, and homeopathic remedies to support their children's health.

Although the topic of vaccination is controversial, I find it important to mention it here. Vaccinations, especially in infants and very young children, are a significant source of toxic exposure that can be damaging to their health. A large portion of the parents I have worked with over the past fifteen years have chosen to either wait, space out, or not vaccinate their children at all due to the harmful effects they can have on certain children. I encourage parents to seek out pediatricians who are open to discussing this topic and do not take a one-size-fits-all approach to your child's health.

Unfortunately, science is imperfect, doctors are unerring, and medical interventions come with risks. While consensus science considers vaccination to be one the greatest inventions in the history of medicine and the greatest achievements of public health programs, the U.S. healthcare system is nearly bankrupt due to the rising cases of chronic inflammatory disease-causing disability. Public health is measured by high vaccination rates and the absence of infectious disease, which does not appear to be moving in the right direction. Most children today receive seventy doses of sixteen federally recommended vaccines. This number has more than doubled since the 1980s, yet statistics show children are sicker than ever.

What I learned very early in my practice is vaccine risks are 100% for *some* children. This is because we are all born equal and alike in the eyes of our Creator, but we are not all born the same. Each of us enters the world with unique genetics, microbiome, and epigenetic influences (birth trauma) that affect how we respond to the environment in which we live. Not a single person on this planet responds the same way to infectious diseases or pharmaceuticals such as vaccines. However, our health care system treats each child (and adults, for that matter) with a standard approach, not considering possible susceptibilities that we may have.

Our healthcare system fails to respect biodiversity and forces everyone to be treated the same, which places a significant risk on a minority of unidentified individuals. Parents who know and love their children better than anyone else want the absolute best for them and trust sound science and concerned public health care policies to help them protect their children from harm. However, if your child's potential susceptibility to a vaccine injury cannot be properly and reliably identified, the child's risk must be pre-determined. Unfortunately, our system has not adopted this way of approaching pharmaceuticals (vaccines). I have worked with parents who have watched the sudden or slow decline of their child's health after routine vaccinations. It has saddened me to watch the amount of time, money, and resources parents spend on things such as heavy metal detoxes, chelation, and different therapies after the fact. Not to mention the ongoing support many of these children will need indefinitely.

My goal is for parents to become aware of the risks and benefits of vaccines before they decide to have children. My desire for the future includes:

- doctors offering informed consent for every single pharmaceutical prescribed,

- prevention of discrimination against vulnerable minorities (many parents have been fired by their pediatrician or criticized for questioning vaccine safety),

- screening for biodiversity in patients before taking a one-size-fits-all approach in medicine and

- establishing parental and human rights with flexible medical, religious, and conscientious belief vaccine exemptions.

Genetics

I have been fascinated with the study of genetics since I was a child. When I was between the ages of 8 and 12, I would walk to a nearby pet store, buy a male and female mouse with specific colors, and take them home. I would then breed them to get a certain look in the babies they would soon have. As I grew older, I dove into the study of epigenetics, which is the study of our genetics and how they can change due to our environment. Before my children were born, I tested my husband and my genetics using basic household test kits. For example, my husband and I both have different MTHFR[iv] which are common genetic mutations that we've passed down to our children. I was aware of this *before* they were born, which enabled me to make choices that would ultimately prevent certain traits associated with MTHFR. These genes can be turned on or off in unborn babies! This knowledge is powerful in preventing disease and ill health within our families. It doesn't necessarily mean you have to run out and test everyone in your family. Still, it does mean that cleaning up your genes by balancing the nervous system, diet, and lifestyle choices will prevent the expression of certain diseases.

The good news is that many parents I've worked with over the last decade have chosen to adopt a cleaner and more intentional way of living. Opting for gluten-free, casein-free meals; no dyes; no refined grains or sugar; removing harmful chemicals from their household and using non-toxic "green" household products; stopping or spacing out vaccinations; using therapeutic-grade essential oils, homeopathic remedies, and supplements as part of a routine to keep their families healthier.

Millions of families now choose to eat healthier organic foods that are chemical-free, take supplements, and even attend yoga classes with their kids. It is absolutely wonderful! This is movement in the right direction! So many parents have taken it upon themselves to learn and educate themselves on healthier ways to raise their children. At the same time, even though a decade does not seem that long, plenty of other factors have changed in the wrong direction, such as stress, fear, and anxiety, which are at an all-time high.

The Third T: Thoughts

The third and final T is about our thoughts. We are more emotionally stressed, busy, revved up, and increasingly over-scheduled than ever before. The Third T (Thoughts) hits families hard, especially these days. Even though many families are improving their lifestyles, stress, fear, and anxiety are at an all-time high. We all need to simplify our lives, but that is easier said than done. Focusing on the basics, such as more quality sleep, healthy meals, entertainment, exercise, and just more family time (without screens), will help us get back to basic human nature. We have so many distractions in our daily lives that we forget to just breathe. My goal with this book is to offer information, alternatives, and resources to help provide healthier options and informed decisions about preconception, pregnancy, and beyond.

WHAT IS FUNCTIONAL MEDICINE?[v]

How do you know if you are truly healthy or not? Maybe you feel fine and are not sick. Unfortunately, feeling fine does not equate to being healthy. Having a trained doctor run the proper tests to identify less-than-optimal functioning in the body is the safest, smartest thing to do prior to conception. Which brings me to Functional Medicine. Functional medicine is for anyone who wants to get to the bottom of a disease rather than continue to subdue the symptoms.

The US healthcare system spends more than 90 percent of its funds on chronic medical conditions with limited success.[vi] It's the biggest healthcare system in the world, amounting to more than $3 trillion per year. Although it provides public health care to around just 20 percent of the population, the rest are dependent on health insurance or paying out-of-pocket. Despite this spending, the US is behind most developed countries when it comes to health care.

There is undoubtedly something wrong with the current healthcare approach that pays enormous attention to acute conditions, relieves symptoms, and provides treatment through various specialists trying to cure the disease of each organ. Modern allopathic[vii] doctors view patients as though they are made of several independent systems.

Functional Medicine (FM) takes a different approach from allopathic. Functional medicine considers a person as a single entity, believing everything is interconnected. It attempts to find the root cause of the ailment, analyzes the potential triggers that led to the present condition, and pays specific attention to the patient's characteristics to provide a personalized remedy and treatment approach.

Functional medicine, the brainchild of Dr. Jeffery Bland, started emerging as one of the branches of alternative medicine in the 1980s. The foundation of functional medicine can be traced back to 1991 when the Institute of Functional Medicine (IFM) was established.

"Functional Medicine is a system. A biology-based approach that focuses on identifying and addressing the root cause of disease. Each symptom or differential diagnosis may be one of many contributing to an individual's illness." – The Functional Medicine Approach, IFM.

Functional medicine attempts to track the origin of the disease, so it pays specific attention to the patient's history. Chronic conditions start much earlier than they are felt and reported, which is something that even allopathy has begun to accept. Now, most researchers recognize that diabetes exists at least a decade before being diagnosed, and the same is true for neurodegenerative diseases. Researchers firmly agree that chronic diseases are the result of a faulty lifestyle practiced for years or even decades. Thus, chronic short duration of sleep may cause hypertension, heart attack, depression, dementia, infertility, and so on.

Despite all the progress and understanding, allopathy rarely tries to correct the root causes, looking instead at the immediate symptoms and alterations in body functions. Thus, drugs are prescribed to control glucose when treating diabetes, and antiseizure medications to keep neuropathy in check. FM is evidence-based medicine with different opinions and outlooks. It sees illness as a reaction or change that occurs due to interaction with the internal and external environments. FM attempts to identify and reverse the ill effects of that interaction by trying to rid the body of the cause and, therefore, cure the system.

Each individual is unique, living and interacting within a unique microenvironment, lifestyle, and influencing factors. The allopathic community understands this, though it does not often take that into consideration when trying to treat diseases. Despite an understanding of the uniqueness of patients, genetics, and environment, allopathy has a "one-size-fits-all" approach.

On the other hand, functional medicine understands that individuals' lifestyle choices and specificity of interaction with the environment play a central role in disease development, modification, and alteration of its course. Interaction with the environment may also change the behavior of the gene, leading to changes in the body: *structural integrity, transport, communication, biotransformation, energy production, defense and repair, and assimilation.* These are the *seven core imbalances* recognized by functional medicine.

To assist the practicing clinicians of functional medicine, the Institute of Functional Medicine (IFM) has developed many innovative tools, including one called the functional medicine matrix[viii], which helps interpret the patient better. Modern research and science help doctors understand the seven core imbalances, thus bridging the knowledge gap. With the help of a matrix, practitioners can better identify the underlying causes (triggers and mediators) of various chronic diseases.

Functional medicine emphasizes four vital components in clinical practice:

1. Carefully listen to and interpret the patient's narrative regarding the ailment and pay specific attention to minute details.

2. Pay attention to modifiable lifestyle factors behind the illness, such as lack of exercise, nutritional deficiencies, lack of sleep, and stress.

3. Complete the matrix table to clarify your understanding of the root causes of diseases.

4. Create a doctor-patient partnership.

Let's look at an example: the doctor-patient collaboration, one of functional medicine's most crucial principles. This principle of partnership has been well studied in the chronic care model of allopathy, yet it is rarely deployed in practice. In allopathy, the doctor prescribes and is in authority, while the patient is expected to fulfill the provided instructions. In functional medicine, the relationship is very different. The doctor and patient are partners in the treatment process.

Functional medicine is not against modern pharmaceutical drugs or allopathic medicine. It complements allopathic medicine, providing the best of various systems. Thus, functional medicine attempts to reverse disease processes through lifestyle modification, exercise, dietary changes, the use of high-quality food supplementation, and even pharmacological drugs. To some extent, functional medicine can be seen as practicing something that allopathic medicine has long talked about but continues to neglect.

Consider, for example, conditions such as dementia, COPD, and diabetes. Most medical texts say treatment should start with identifying the root cause, followed by lifestyle modification. Yet, in actual practice, allopathic doctors rarely do that; instead, they immediately begin treatment with proven—or even unproven—drugs.

In functional medicine, treatment starts with fundamental changes in lifestyle, nutritional interventions, and prioritizing the correction of the seven core imbalances. Ultimately, it results in a better quality of life, better outcomes, and reduced health care costs, with or without minimal use of any toxic therapies.

Another emphasis of functional medicine is on the so-called therapeutic relationship. The qualities of trust, gratitude, vulnerability, presence, humility, deep listening, reflection, and connection are considered essential to the healing process. It is vital to understand the patient's preparedness to change. Outcomes depend significantly on the practitioner's ability to motivate patients to comply with lifestyle prescriptions and to make necessary changes, thus allowing the body to begin correcting underlying imbalances.

One of the greatest strengths of functional medicine is that its principles can be applied with equal success to all the disciplines and specialties of medicine. The template of the functional medicine matrix can be utilized to understand the patient and the root causes of diseases and in planning the therapeutic approach. Functional medicine combines various components of traditional and nontraditional medicine to treat, prevent, and reverse chronic diseases.

Though allopathic medicine practitioners agree with many underlying principles of functional medicine—identifying the root cause, lifestyle modifications, stress management, and nutrition therapy—most are skeptical about many tenets of functional medicine. Many practitioners of allopathy are skeptical about the methods that correct the flow of vital energy, techniques to help activate and deactivate genes during development (gene switching), and detoxification. The reason for this skepticism is often their lack of awareness and understanding of some of the latest findings in research.

Most allopathic doctors would say switching genes on and off is impossible to cure ailments. However, those who state this forget about (or need to be made aware of) the field in modern science called epigenetics, the study of heritable phenotype changes that do not involve alterations in the DNA sequence. Epigenetics most often involves changes that affect gene activity and expression. Such effects on cellular and physiological phenotypic traits may result from external or environmental factors or be part of normal development. The standard definition of epigenetics requires these alterations to be heritable in the progeny of either cells or organisms. Epigenetics says that with lifestyle modification, it is possible to change gene expression. Stated, lifestyle changes may help to switch individual genes on and off. Moreover, the study of epigenetics (also part of allopathy) confirms that such changes can be passed on to the next generation.

Correction of energy flow (bioenergy) is another area that practitioners of allopathy may discount. However, it is something entirely supported by science. It is now well known that nerves and hormones control the functioning of every cell in our body. Without nerve supply, many cells would die immediately.

Functional medicine recommends looking at the body as a single entity, not something comprised of independent systems. Modern science is now proving that various bodily systems are more related to each other than ever thought before. We have all heard about—and probably experienced—a "gut feeling," which occurs because our gut has more neurons than the spine, and these neurons secrete hundreds of hormones, neurohormones, and neurotransmitters. In recent years, scholars have coined the term "diffuse endocrine system" because they realized that hormones are released by almost all the tissues and not just by the traditional endocrine organs. It has been well-proven that even fat tissue around a person's midsection secretes several hormones that have a role in health and disease development.

Many practitioners of allopathy are also skeptical about reversing chronic ailments, even though there are many examples of this being done. Moreover, in the last few decades, it has been established that under specific conditions, every organ has the capacity to recover and regenerate. Stem-cell therapy and regenerative medicine started by identifying the super-regenerative powers of particular tissues, such as bone marrow or embryonic stem cells. Now, it is recognized beyond doubt that stem cells—which can regenerate—exist in all tissues and organs.

Much of the skepticism regarding functional medicine is due to a need for more awareness and/or neglect of long-proven principles of modern health science. The diagnostic approach in functional medicine differs significantly from allopathic medicine. Functional medicine focuses on disease prevention by identifying the root cause, unlike allopathic medicine, where tests are usually done to confirm a diagnosis. Thus, in allopathic medicine, doctors order a test to confirm the pathological changes and diagnosis. In contrast, the doctor's goal in functional medicine is to learn more about conditions such as leaky gut syndrome, infections, food intolerance, and hormonal and nutrient deficiencies, not just to search for some inflammatory markers that indicate a disease process.

For example, functional medicine doctors often order a comprehensive stool test to learn how the digestive system is working and about the levels of good and bad bacteria in the gut. This determines the presence of highly virulent infections and how a person absorbs various nutrients. In a blood test, doctors of functional medicine are interested in nutritional deficiencies that may lead to depression, fibromyalgia, sleep disturbances, diabetes, and fatigue, unlike allopathic doctors who are more interested in markers of inflammation and infection.

Doctors of functional medicine are also greatly interested in the complete hormonal profile. They pay attention to the adrenal stress profile, as these hormones are the most significant indicators of acute or chronic stress, which is behind the development of various diseases. Often, it is hormonal changes, chronic stress, and inflammation that lead to autoimmune disorders.

Other tests that doctors of functional medicine will order are a detailed cardiometabolic profile and tests for heavy metals and chemical toxins. Doctors of functional medicine also look deeper into food sensitivities.

So, who should consult with a functional medicine doctor, and for what health issues and diseases does it work best?

Allopathic medicine is excellent at acute care, meaning if you were having severe pain in your abdomen along with vomiting and diarrhea, you wouldn't want to see a functional medicine doctor. You would need acute care, or you could die of your appendix rupturing. Functional medicine is about disease prevention, finding the root causes of chronic health challenges or diseases, detoxification, metabolism correction, and disease reversal.

Think about it like this: if a person had a heart attack, allopathic medicine could help to save a life, but once the condition has stabilized, functional medicine can help to identify the causes of worsening cardiac health, high blood pressure, high cholesterol; it can help to correct the faulty lifestyle and assist in disease reversal. Functional medicine can be beneficial in the treatment of diabetes, asthma, food allergies, celiac disease, autoimmune diseases, mood disorders, and much more.

Functional medicine is for anyone who wants to get to the bottom of the disease rather than continue to subdue the symptoms.

PRECONCEPTION: PREPARING FOR BABY

You can do so much to prepare your body for pregnancy, and when you do, you help ensure you and your future baby are as healthy as possible. Finding a neurologically trained chiropractor, functional medicine practitioner, naturopath, nutritionist, dietician, acupuncturist, osteopath, or someone knowledgeable in this area will greatly benefit you on this journey. Physicians trained in this field can run proper functional tests and assessments to identify any less-than-optimal functioning in the body, and they can help correct those issues before you conceive your child. Being proactive in this way with your health greatly reduces the chances of chronic health issues in children and postpartum mothers and ensures healthier generations to come.

Pre-pregnancy care (also called preconception care) addresses not only the mother's physical health (ideally, both parents are assessed since it takes Mom and Dad to make a baby) but also her mental and emotional health. Different issues within this realm may be best handled by a trained psychiatrist.

If you are hoping to become pregnant soon or have been trying for some time, here are some tips that can help you prepare your body, mind, and soul for the journey of bringing life into the world.

Neurological Chiropractic:

First and foremost, have your nervous system assessed by a chiropractor. This step cannot be overstated enough. If your nervous system is not in balance due to the 3-T's (Trauma, Toxicity, Thoughts) and if you have subluxations as a result, you will have a much harder time achieving optimal health for both you and your unborn child. When your brain, nervous system, and Vagus nerve communicate properly with all the cells in your body, you will experience more success with changing your diet, getting more quality sleep, exercise, and supplementation.

Clean Up Your Diet:

When preparing for pregnancy, the most important thing you can do is remove unhealthy food from your diet and replace it with healthy foods and balanced meals. I look at it like this: a gardener always nourishes the soil as much as they can before they plant the precious seeds—the healthier the soil, the more vibrantly those seeds will grow. Our bodies are similar. The healthier we are physically before pregnancy, the better the environment to maintain a healthy pregnancy: Eat organic, hormone-free, GMO-free, whole foods that nourish you. Make sure to get an ample amount of protein from clean sources as well.

The following information reviews the best ways to supplement during preconception and pregnancy.

Supplement Appropriately (in addition to a healthy, well-rounded diet and lifestyle):

In the following suggestions, the recommended amounts to be taken are to support preconception, the prenatal period, and breastfeeding mothers. You should always consult with a trained physician before taking any supplement.

Your prenatal multivitamin should contain ACTIVE B vitamins and other key nutrients to build a healthy baby. DO NOT buy your prenatal from a big-box retailer; the quality is not there. Also, it is not a good idea to get a prescription prenatal vitamin from your doctor (even though they are free in most cases). These prescriptions contain synthetic, nonactive vitamins, including folic acid (which will be explained later), and artificial coloring.

NOTE – some nutrients listed below may be found in your prenatal vitamin. In that case, lesser amounts of these nutrients below may be needed.

- **Active B12 (methylcobalamin) is needed for crucial functions, such as the formation of red blood cells, energy production, the** nervous system, and cognitive support. Make sure your B12 is always "active" or methylated. I recommend a minimum of 1,000 mcg daily. Methylcobalamin is naturally found in red meat.

- **Active folate (methyl folate)** supports cellular methylation and is crucial for those with MTHFR genetic mutation.

(Folic acid has been shown to be toxic to people with this defect and leads to increased chances of midline defects in the unborn baby if the mother ingests this while pregnant.) **L-methylfolate, also known as 5-MTHF**, is the active form of vitamin B9 that the human body can use. (Folic acid is synthetic and therefore nonactive and not usable by most people.) This nutrient is needed to form healthy cells, especially red blood cells, and it protects against neural tube defects. The amount needed varies greatly per person, but it is recommended to start off very low (1 mg) and work up as needed. Working with a trained physician is very important. Active folate is naturally found in green, leafy vegetables.

- **Vitamin D3/K2** should be in a pure base of olive oil or coconut oil. Vitamin D protects your immune system as well as so many other systems and functions in the body. We North Americans are some of the most deficient in this important nutrient. While pregnant, breastfeeding, and trying to become pregnant, it is recommended to take a minimum of 6,500 IU daily. Have your doctor monitor your vitamin D levels every three months.

- **Probiotics** are very important supplements because most of us do not get them through our diet. Probiotics are beneficial bacteria that improve the immune and gut health of both mother and baby. Probiotics are best absorbed with the evening meal. You can also get naturally occurring probiotics in fermented foods such as sauerkraut, kimchi, kefir, and kombucha.

- **Calcium/magnesium** must be taken together to be absorbed properly. Calcium citrate, calcium malate, and calcium bisglycinate chelate are the most absorbable forms. Having enough calcium in your body is essential to protect your unborn child from lead absorption. If the mother is deficient in calcium, the baby's body will pull calcium out of her bones and deposit it into theirs, subsequently pulling lead along with it, leading to lead absorption. I recommend 800 mg daily during preconception, pregnancy, and breastfeeding.

- **Fish oil that provides the proper amount of EPA/DHA in the triglyceride form** is better absorbed than the ethyl ester form. Ample fish oils help form the baby's growing brain and nervous system and protect the mother's cognitive health. A minimum of 1,000 mg daily is recommended with a proper 2:1 EPA to DHA ratio. Choose the healthiest fish your budget can afford, ideally wild-caught salmon, to make sure you are also getting naturally occurring EPA/DHA while also avoiding high amounts of mercury.

- **Choline** is a common deficiency in pregnant and breastfeeding mothers. This is very important as choline is a critical nutrient in cognitive development. It is a fact that only 15 percent of women have adequate choline levels.

Supplementing with high-quality choline is important, as well as getting it in our diet through beef liver, eggs, seafood, meats, flax seeds, Brussels sprouts, and broccoli. When supplementing, 800 mg daily is recommended.

- Optimal amounts of **healthy protein** are also recommended during preconception, pregnancy, and breastfeeding. Ideally, one gram per pound of ideal body weight is a great measure to live by. Keeping in mind what your total calorie goal is, depending on the weight you want to maintain, lose, or gain, that amount can fluctuate between 0.7 to 1.0 grams per pound body weight (referenced from Dr Gabrielle Lyons). Pregnant and breastfeeding women need at minimum one hundred grams of protein daily, ideally more, and exclusively breastfeeding mothers need a minimum of seventy grams per day. Choose between a variety of red meat, meat sticks, chicken, eggs, kefir, or Greek yogurt (as long as you're not intolerant to dairy). Some vegetarian options are hemp seeds and lentil soup. If you're like me and have a hard time getting enough protein, you can supplement with a scoop of collagen protein throughout your day.

Go Gluten-Free[ix]

There is growing evidence that gluten intolerance is less of a fad than we thought. In fact, these infamous proteins, gliadin and glutenin, can wreak havoc on a person's bodily systems and general health. Unfortunately, many people consume ordinary foods that contain this protein daily, unaware of the adverse reactions gluten has on their systems. Anyone who chooses to munch daily on a burger, fries, and soda is shortening their lifespan, but even if they have a big slice of whole-wheat bread instead (a healthier option), there can still be negative consequences.

Wheat and other cereals like rye, barley, spelt, and oats, as well as processed and boxed meals, contain gluten. In the average Western diet, it's also found in bread, pizzas, pies, and pasta. Furthermore, the types of wheat found in the US are fortified with higher levels of gluten to make bread and breadlike products fluffy and puffy.

Gluten has been a component of human nutrition for ages. It gives us the energy and stamina we need to go through the day and makes us feel full and happy. The question that should be asked, then, is this: Why do so many of us have gluten intolerance if this is what we've been consuming every day for years? There are numerous reasons for this, including genetic predisposition and, specifically, an insufficient ability to metabolize grains and grass. Wheat first entered Europe during the medieval times, and 30 percent of European ancestors are genetically predisposed to celiac disease, which raises the risk of developing a health issue because of gluten consumption.

More of the healthier foods we consume have been contaminated with gluten, including corn and oatmeal. Not only that but it's also found in product ingredients like malt and maltodextrin, which is why reading product labels is so important.

The most shocking evidence, though, is that 99 percent of people with a gluten intolerance are unaware they have it, so they fail to blame their poor health on their gluten intolerance. As someone who works with people daily to address and improve their health concerns, this is very disappointing and challenging because the symptoms that come from gluten intolerance are 100 percent treatable.

Gluten intolerance is typically connected with two triggers: genetic predisposition and intestinal permeability or leaky gut. In the first case, being gluten sensitive does not imply that you are a sensitive person. It just means that your DNA and immune system cannot tolerate gluten. Your immune system may falsely flag it as a foreign intruder and attempt to attack it. In essence, this is what "gluten sensitivity" means. Fortunately, you can easily be tested for gluten sensitivity and learn whether you have these genetic tendencies.

Get Healthy Exercise

The right amount of exercise (not too much and not too little) does wonders for your mood, energy, hormonal balance, and overall health. Getting exercise early in the day is better than exercising late in the evening. If you exercise later in the day, make sure it is light exercise so that it does not interfere with your sleep circadian rhythm (sleep cycles).

Committing to Your Fitness

Similar to discussing your menstrual cycle during fitness, as soon as you achieve pregnancy, people around you may start discouraging you from staying on your fitness and training journey. Some pregnant women are told all the things they can no longer do because they are seemingly "fragile." That has always struck a cord in me. Many women in my practice are told to stop exercising, limit exercise, or change their training schedule. This is, of course, going to happen naturally when/if the fatigue sets in during the first trimester. However, there is no reason for you to stop your exercising and training routine if you are healthy and feeling well. I like to think about all the things you CAN do instead of discussing the activities you CAN'T. Obviously, if you haven't been training for a marathon and you get pregnant, it's going to be a really bad idea to start training for one at that time. The only thing that makes us fragile is NOT having a fitness and exercise routine. Being sedentary before you get pregnant is going to cause a more difficult pregnancy in general, so there's no better time than the present moment to commit to your health and start moving! It is one of the greatest gifts you can give yourself. One of the best ways to do this is through exercise. It takes time and dedication, but the results are always worth it. Exercise has proven benefits that can impact anyone at any stage of life in a positive way. Just a few of the health benefits of exercise include:

- Improved Mood
- Weight Loss
- Prevent Osteoporosis
- More Energy
- Better Sleep
- Reduced risk of disease
- Decreased stress
- Improved memory

When it comes to chronic disease, exercise is also a win-win. Working out is known for improving insulin sensitivity while decreasing blood pressure and blood fat levels.[x] Lack of exercise creates excess belly fat and is attributed to heart disease, obesity, type 2 diabetes, as well as early death. Therefore, daily exercise is recommended to combat belly fat, maintain a healthy body weight, and decrease the risk of these diseases for a healthy immune system.

The heart also needs to be exercised like a muscle to function properly. When the heart works effectively, it can pull more oxygen out of the blood to decrease the pumping of blood to surrounding muscles and work harder. This helps reduce the chance of stress hormones putting more pressure on the heart, working as a beta-blocker to lower blood pressure and slow the heart rate. Aerobic exercise, also known as cardiovascular exercise, is the best exercise for your heart.

Exercise is known to improve brain health by increasing the blood flow from the heart to the brain through cardiovascular stimulation. The faster and harder your heart beats when you exercise, the more oxygen will also be pumped to the brain. This means elevating your heart rate has a positive impact on your brain performance and can help your memory as you get older.[xi]

Being physically active can also help improve digestion, which is something many people struggle with. During exercise, more blood is being produced throughout the body and flows toward the digestive system. This can help to relieve symptoms of gas, bloating, heartburn, cramps, and constipation.[xii] In general, your organs are more efficient when you're in shape!

Finally, exercise makes you feel good! A variety of hormones are secreted when you work out. These are known as endorphins. Your brain secretes more dopamine and serotonin, which are known as the happiness chemicals. Additionally, over time, exercise also helps to decrease your cortisol levels, which is the stress hormone. Cortisol is often released in "fight or flight" mode, so the body feels stressed which later causes disease. However, too much exercise can also be counterintuitive.

Breathing

How often do you think about your breath? If you're like anyone else, probably not that much! Breathing is a vital process of the body that is directly linked to the overall performance of our body and brain. We breathe 15x/minute or 21,000 times per day![xiii] This means when we exercise, breathing is important!

The process of respiration, also known as breathing, burns glucose and oxygen in the body so that muscular contractions, mental processes, and glandular secretions occur. If you want your body to be in peak performance for exercise, it's time to take note of how you breathe, not only regularly, but also when working out.

Many people breathe incorrectly, which results in shallow breathing. This means they're not using their full lung capacity, and the body is deprived of the essential oxygen that it needs to function optimally. When you use your full lung capacity, you use your diaphragm to breathe. Your diaphragm is your breathing muscle centered between your chest and your abdomen. When you inhale, it contracts to bring air in, and when you exhale, it relaxes to release air out.

Slow, deep breaths are associated with calm and content states of mind. Irregular and fast-paced breathing indicates anxiety or panic. The way this works is through the nervous system. Our breath is an amazing tool we can use because we can control it, unlike other automatic processes such as the heartbeat or digestion. Many animals that breathe slower also live longer, like elephants and turtles. Animals with shallow, quick breaths live shorter lives, like rodents and dogs.

The breath can be very helpful when performing difficult movements, such as pullups or lifting heavy weights like bench pressing. In this case, it is best to use the exhale on exertion, as it is the more powerful part of the breath. For example, when you perform a pullup, you will exhale on the way up and inhale as you lower down.

Foundation of Core Movement

When most people think of the core, the first thing that comes to mind is the abdominals. Everyone wants defined abs, but beyond that, strong abdominals can prevent injury and overall assist movement.

However, the core is comprised of 3 areas, not just the award-winning ab area. In addition to the abdominals, the core is also made up of the hips and lower back, which are all linked together. These three areas work in sync to stabilize the center of the body.

Most core movement relies on the principle of the midline. The midline is not only the physical spine but also an imaginary line through the center of the body. The theory goes that most movement is more efficient when you pull it into toward the center or the midline. So, to find stronger movement, one must streamline their effort by contracting the muscles into the midline to go further, faster, push higher or harder, etc. This is like a rebound effect. Think of a coil- it contracts backward only to propel itself further forward.

A general rule of thumb to activate the core or engage the abdominals is to brace the core by pulling the abdomen in. You can think of the abdomen as an abdominal scoop that lifts inward toward the spine. This helps to not only protect all of the organs in the area but also promote blood flow and protect the back muscles and skeletal structure of the hips and spine.

The abdominal scooping action helps to activate the deep core muscles, which go beyond the superficial six-pack. These deep core muscles stabilize the trunk of the body.

Many people often complain they have thrown their back out when picking up a heavy object off the floor. This is a combination of poor lifting posture and weak abdominal muscles. Strong deep core muscles are so important because they help prevent this common lifting injury by bracing the spine in combination with the proper technique of bending the knees to lift something heavy.

Low Impact Exercise

Some people dread exercise because of the thought of getting sore or causing injury. If you're recovering from an injury or have a health condition that prevents you from an intense workout, low-impact exercise is the solution. It's also a great way to ease back into an exercise routine if you have been out for a while.

Low-impact exercise still elevates the heart rate, burns fat, and tones muscles without putting as much stress on the body as running, skiing, or gymnastics. These types of exercise put you more at risk for injury. Walking, cycling, and yoga are all great recommendations for low-impact exercise.

Walking

If you have two feet, use them! Walking is a free and easy exercise you can do anytime, anywhere. Go for a walk outside in your neighborhood, through a local park, or even in a big shopping mall if it's too hot or cold outside. Get some good walking shoes for support and hit the pavement!

Yoga

The physical health benefits of yoga are undeniable and practiced by millions worldwide. There are many different styles that cater to various needs. Vinyasa, Ashtanga, or power yoga are great workouts as they are more intense with constant flowing movement. Hatha yoga also strengthens; however, the postures are held for longer periods, so it's excellent for developing balance and stability. Other types of yoga, such as yin or restorative yoga, are also great because they emphasize long holds in reclined or seated postures that allow for a deep stretch. Stretching is an important part of fitness that many forget!

If you work your muscles regularly into a contracted state through intense physical exercise, they also need to be released to prevent soreness and improve the range of motion in the joints. All styles of yoga can help with this, not to mention the added benefit it has on the state of mind, too.

Yoga is also not just stretching; it utilizes the breath to create a bridge between the body and the mind to allow for a deeper experience that is often very healing for many people. It is loved by many as a form of exercise that can prevent injuries when done correctly in proper alignment and help some recover from injuries.

Cycling

Cycling is yet another great, low-impact form of exercise. This can also be done outdoors or indoors on a stationary bike. Cycling is a great alternative to running as it does not stress the knees or ankles as running can nor tighten the hamstrings or lower back the way running does. It still moves the body at regular intervals to get the heart rate up to burn fat and keep the heart healthy. It is a great exercise regimen for people with trouble with their knees or tight hamstrings.

Resistance Training

Resistance training is a way to build your endurance and overall muscular strength. Types of equipment include weights, dumbbells, exercise bands, bars, and even gravity. You may also use medicine balls, kettlebells, or weight machines at the gym.

Generally, resistance training is considered a safe alternative to weight training as it is gentler on the joints. Resistance training will burn fat and tone muscle, while weight training can put you at risk for injury due to the greater range of motion required.

As a form of strength training, resistance training should be performed 2-3 times per week to see results. It can also be done every day. There are over 600 muscles in the human body, so you can spread the target areas over a week or a few days. Different workouts and equipment will target different muscle groups. You can alternate muscle groups daily for the whole body to get toned effectively. For example, in a 3-day workout plan, you can plan to do legs on Day 1, upper body on Day 2, and then the whole body on Day 3.

Examples of resistance training exercises include barbell squats, biceps curls, pull-ups, and rowing to give you an idea. TRX, using suspension straps, is another great form of resistance exercise that uses gravity and your body weight to achieve a workout.

Flexibility

The age-old saying goes, "You are only as young as your spine is flexible." While you don't need to be a contortionist to be flexible, there are many health benefits that flexibility offers, such as:

- Improved posture
- Recovery from injury
- Decreased physical pain and muscular soreness
- Better balance and coordination
- More strength
- A positive outlook on life

Flexibility is gained by stretching. When you stretch, you bring more blood flow and oxygen into the muscles. If there is any damage or injuries, this will help nourish and repair the muscular fibers. Stretching can improve your overall physical performance ability by allowing your muscles to work more effectively and in a greater range of motion. If the muscles are tight and contracted and stress is placed on them, the risk of injury is higher. Stretching is an essential part of any exercise regimen!

In athletic performance, flexibility is also vital when it comes to speed. For example, a runner who does not incorporate a stretching routine will have less strength and power in their muscles to fire quickly, so the chance of injury grows.

For most, flexibility is merely a physical practice of moving the joints and muscles through their full range of motion. However, flexibility can also be a state of mind. As stretching releases tension from the body, you can also think of it as relieving tension in the mind. Therefore, stretching can bring peace of mind and help us deal with difficult situations more easily.

Posture

Believe it or not, your posture also plays a role in your overall health. Many daily aches and pains, such as lower back pain, are often attributed to poor posture. Your posture is essentially the position you hold your body in while sitting or standing. What we call good posture is when the bones and joints are in alignment to support the proper functioning of the muscles. This means that when you have good posture, the muscles can work more efficiently, use less energy, and become less fatigued, which we can measure using **Insight Technology!**

It is important to develop an awareness of your posture to correct anything that may be causing harm. For example, a common postural imbalance is forward head posture or loss of the cervical lordosis. We see this in almost every adult starting care in our office. The sad reality is that many of us were not breastfed or were not breastfed long enough for the neck and jaw muscles to develop with enough strength to allow for a strong cervical spine to support the cranium. As a result, the neck weakens, and the head falls forward, creating a whole host of postural distortions in the spine.

The cranium and pelvis are designed to be stacked, one over the other, to create a more stable spinal structure. Unfortunately, when the cranium develops in a forward posture, over time, the pelvis also follows and more in a forward position as well. This condition is a tilted pelvis that places pressure on the discs and joints of the lower back.

Some may think that if there is pain in the body, not to exercise. But the truth is, exercise often helps to treat and prevent not only injuries but also postural conditions. Through core conditioning and spinal exercises, lumbar lordosis can be treated and corrected to alleviate painful symptoms.

The same can be said for another common misalignment: slouching or computer/cell phone posture, which causes the shoulders to slump forward. You can bring awareness to this by correcting your posture when you sit as a static postural exercise. Dynamic posture is how you hold your body when you exercise. Through specific exercises and stretches, the muscles in the area can be released so that your old posture is replaced by a new posture that healthily supports your body.

Healthy posture makes us feel better and can display several benefits, such as more confidence, increased lung capacity, and a stronger spine.

It is vital to connect your breath to your posture and every movement you make. Our breath is like the language in which we can communicate with our bodies. Remember this whenever you exercise and notice the difference in your workout, posture, and mindset.

Sleep

Getting enough sleep is important for all beings to function properly. When we do not get our required amount of sleep each night, we are not giving our bodies the opportunity to heal and repair. When trying to conceive, make sure you aim to get into bed by 10:30 p.m. at the latest and to wake seven to nine hours later, depending on your need for rest. This helps heal and repair your body, and it also helps you overcome hormonal challenges.

Know Your Cycle

When you count your cycle, always start on the first day of your period, which is Day One. If you have a twenty-eight-day cycle, the fertile window is normally two weeks before your next suspected period, so that would be around Day Fourteen. Often, women's cycles are all different lengths. Some women have twenty-one-day cycles (or shorter), and others have cycles that are forty-five days or longer. A cycle that is too short or too long may affect fertility. Talking with your alternative provider and getting the appropriate hormonal testing done to identify why your cycle length is too long or too short could be helpful. Several apps are available that help women keep track of their cycle, as well as document symptoms that come with the change in hormones.

Trust Divine Timing

Nothing is more frustrating than wanting something so badly that is not happening when you want it to. For some, becoming pregnant happens right away, while it takes others some time. All beings have their divine timing; just because you are ready to have a baby does not mean that this child is ready to come into the world just yet. If you can surrender and trust Divine timing, you will come to understand the reason that things do not always happen when you want them to. In time, answers will always be revealed.

Make Better Health Choices Before Conception

Preconception care is an opportunity for you and your partner to improve your health before you bring a new life into this world. It takes both mother and father to produce a high-quality sperm and egg, resulting in a new life with robust health. A neurologically trained chiropractor can assess the state of your overall nervous system and an alternative health-care professional can help you assess your health, fitness, and lifestyle, as well as identify areas that you may want to improve. Allow plenty of time for preconception planning and care before you start trying to conceive.

You may ask, "Why is this so important?" You will increase your chances of getting pregnant if you and your partner are in good health. A poor diet, being overweight or obese, smoking, drinking, high stress, poor-quality sleep, and unhealthy working conditions can affect the quality of sperm and stop you from becoming pregnant. Ideally, both partners try to make your lifestyle as healthy as possible before you try to conceive.

PREGNANCY AND CHIROPRACTIC

The topic of birth is near and dear to my heart because of my passion for helping pregnant mothers birth their babies naturally. I've been enamored with birth ever since I was present for the births of my younger sisters. My mother was fortunate to bring all of us into this world naturally and in the comfort of our home. Being the oldest, I was by her side each time. From the moment I was able to witness the power of birth, I was amazed by the capabilities of a woman's body. I knew someday, if I were to bring children into this world, I would want to do it the way my empowered mother did.

Today, the focus of my work is to educate and empower women considering pregnancy and to support all expectant mothers by helping their bodies stay strong and balanced so that they can birth the way their bodies are meant to. Supporting women in this way is one of the greatest feelings—and one of the many reasons I love what I do.

PREGNANCY, LABOR AND DELIVERY WITH CHIROPRACTIC

Having a baby is one of the most important decisions a woman will make in her lifetime, and for the most part, the healthiest possible outcome is determined by the choices she and her partner make. Pregnancy is a time of tremendous change in the body, from conception to birth and afterward. While the growing abdomen and posture changes are the most obvious transformations, countless hormonal and chemical shifts occur within the mother and the developing child as well. Chiropractic care may help alleviate the extra burden placed on the spine, while contributing to a responsive, fully functional nervous system.

The noninvasive health care and maintenance provided by specific neurological chiropractic adjustments are absolutely beneficial to the general population, but they may be of particular value to pregnant women. Pregnancy produces hormones that relax the ligaments to allow for childbirth, while the growing belly shifts a woman's center of gravity, increasing vulnerability to spinal misalignment and injury. Chiropractic care can help align spinal and soft-tissue structures, as well as benefit the greater health and well-being of mother and baby.

In addition, chiropractic supports the body by making it stronger, as well as more flexible and balanced before conception, which can promote a more regular menstrual cycle and optimize uterine function. Students in chiropractic college take courses in obstetrics and pediatrics to gain knowledge and understanding for their future patients. Regular chiropractic care also improves hormonal- and immune-system functions in a very natural way by promoting proper nervous system communication from the brain to the body's vital organs.

Studies suggest chiropractic care results in easier labor and delivery for an overall healthier pregnancy (Fallon, J, DC. Chiropractic and Pregnancy. New York: New Rochelle 1998). Pelvic alignment is also important to ensure the baby has enough room to shift into the correct position for proper growth and development. Chiropractic care may also increase the mother's comfort during labor and delivery, reducing the need for analgesics and leading to significantly shorter labor times.

A misaligned pelvis may result in less intrauterine room in her pelvis, making it difficult for the baby to have ample room for growth and development, as well as getting into the best possible position for delivery. To provide a chiropractic adjustment to a pregnant woman's body, special tables and pillows are used to help her avoid excessive pressure on her abdomen. The Webster Technique, which I will cover in detail, was developed to establish greater balance in the pelvic region and to reduce stress on supporting ligaments of the pelvis. It helps malpositioned babies (babies that are posterior, oblique, transverse, or breech) find balance within the womb so that they may naturally find the correct position for themselves. After birth, a postnatal chiropractic examination and adjustments of the mother's spine and soft-tissue structures may help the new mother in many ways, including less pain, better posture, increased milk production, easier breastfeeding, faster healing and recovery, more energy, less fatigue, and reduced chances of postpartum depression.

HOW CAN CHIROPRACTIC CARE HELP ME DURING MY PREGNANCY, LABOR, AND DELIVERY?

Should pregnant women undergo chiropractic care? This is an important question, and all pregnant women should understand that prenatal chiropractic is safe, natural, and effective. In my opinion, all women considering becoming pregnant, as well as those who are pregnant or postnatal, should seek out chiropractic care. During pregnancy, a woman's body undergoes many physiological, structural, hormonal, and emotional changes as the baby inside the womb begins to grow and develop. Due to these changes, the pregnant mother experiences various forms of misalignments in her joints and spine that result in one or a combination of the following:

- A growing, prominent curve of the lower back
- Enlargement of the breasts and abdomen resulting in flattened ribs and increased stress on the thoracic spine
- Pelvic shifts and changes
- Postural changes, including forward head posture

These changes in the pregnant woman's body could result in the female experiencing difficulty attaining proper balance and alignment. Chiropractic care helps the woman's body correct and adapt to these conditions and enables the development of better posture that places less stress on the pregnant body. As previously discussed, the misalignment of a pregnant woman's pelvis could restrict or limit the growing, developing baby inside the womb.

CHIROPRACTIC BENEFITS FOR THE PREGNANT WOMEN

Pregnancy should be a very exciting time in a woman's life, yet it can be overshadowed by extreme pain and discomfort. This occurs because, during pregnancy, women undergo tremendous structural and hormonal changes that affect the nerves, spine, ligaments, organs, and even their overall stability. A doctor of chiropractic can help the spinal column, pelvis, and all related structures move properly, stay balanced, and remain free from vertebral subluxation and nerve interference.

All licensed chiropractors are trained in using chiropractic procedures on pregnant women, and there are chiropractic professionals who specialize in treatments for prenatal and postnatal care (as our office does). These professionals are required to complete hundreds of hours of postgraduate training to direct their specialization to ensure the safety of both baby and mother.

Chiropractors who treat pregnant women must adjust the intensity of their treatment procedures, depending on on the woman's condition and the stage of her gestation period. Many times, chiropractors will recommend a regimen of stretching and exercise to be done at home to ensure optimum effectiveness of chiropractic care and therefore optimal health of the mother and child.

Before women undergo labor, it is highly recommended that they undergo chiropractic care as it assists in many ways throughout pregnancy and delivery. The following is a list of health benefits that result from having chiropractic care during pregnancy as it:

- helps achieve an overall healthier pregnancy.

- enables the patient to maintain control over symptoms and conditions associated with pregnancy.

- enables the patient to have a more efficient, effective delivery.

- relieves pain in the neck, back, and joints, which undergo tremendous strain during pregnancy.

- helps to reduce stress in mom and baby during labor and delivery and reduces the total labor and delivery time.

- allows the spine, hips, and pelvis to be more flexible.

- provides a drug-free alternative. The more medicine a pregnant woman takes, the higher the chances of damaging her baby and her own body.

- helps prevent the need for intervention—forceps, vacuum, or Cesarean section (C-section) delivery. With these types of delivery, the risk of complications for mom and baby is greatly increased, especially with a C-section.

- makes the mother more physically comfortable (after delivery) during breastfeeding and aids in the production of breast milk.
- helps decrease the chances of having (or eliminates) any form of back labor contractions and sharp pain felt in the lower back during labor.

CHIROPRACTIC EFFECTS DURING LABOR

In addition to the benefits of prenatal conditions mentioned above, chiropractic care offers great benefits during the actual labor and delivery of the baby, especially in terms of pain management. Many women who receive chiropractic care throughout their pregnancy and during labor report a more successful delivery.

When the human body undergoes the extremely stressful situation of delivering a baby, the balance and adaptability of the pregnant woman's body is crucial. Most women who undergo a Cesarean section must do so because of the body's inability to cope with the normal stress of delivery. Many times, a woman must deliver via C-section because of a misalignment of the pelvis, which slows down the descent of the baby toward the birth canal. Additionally, limited range of motion in the woman's lower back and hips is also a culprit that affects a woman's ability to labor efficiently. Hence, receiving chiropractic adjustments during pregnancy, enables a woman to address the above problems and may significantly reduce her time in labor. I will elaborate on the physical benefits of chiropractic adjustments later in the chapter.

Another component that impacts labor time is the positioning of the baby. Chiropractic treatments can help the baby find a natural balance in their position and alignment within the mother's womb. Toward the end of the third trimester, this enables the baby to have its head placed directly upon the mother's cervix, which allows for more efficient dilation and, therefore, shortened labor times.

WHAT DO I LOOK FOR IN A CHIROPRACTOR IF I'M PREGNANT?

Prenatal chiropractic care, or chiropractic care for pregnant women, is an important, frequently used service chiropractors provide. All chiropractors are trained to manage the unique set of neuromusculoskeletal symptoms that arise during pregnancy and to improve the mother's quality of life. Some chiropractors, however, specialize in this discipline and provide personalized care to women before, during, and after their pregnancy.

An important thing to keep in mind is that while every chiropractor has been trained to treat all types of patients, including pregnant women, it may be an even better experience to find a chiropractor who has extra training or who specializes in treating pregnant women. These physicians have more experience and know more ways to help the pregnant mother since this was their focus during college and in postgraduate studies. They are more sensitive to the needs of both the patient and the growing child, which can make it an easier, more effective experience.

If chiropractic during your pregnancy is so important, how do you find a chiropractor who knows how to work with pregnant women? To find chiropractors who specialize in and who have received extra training to work with pregnant women appropriately and safely, please visit www.icpa4kids.

org to find a trained chiropractor near you. If you look for ICPA practitioners in your area and none are available, the next best course of action is to talk to local birth professionals. Midwives and doulas often recommend chiropractors who they have found get good results, helping their mothers have more comfortable pregnancies and births. Your childbirth educator, as well as other birthing women in your area, may also have some good suggestions.

Seeking out a skilled doctor of chiropractic to assist you throughout your pregnancy is a must on your list of labor preparations. Some chiropractors are open to visits during labor, which can provide relief as well as miraculous results. I encourage women who are preparing for a natural birth to become as educated as they can on natural birth so that they have an in-depth understanding of what their body can do. Educating ourselves in this way optimizes our chances of a safe, natural, healthy delivery, as well as brings us peace of mind and a better experience overall.

SHOULD I HAVE A CHIROPRACTOR ON MY BIRTH TEAM?

If you are pregnant, one of the best things you can do for you and your baby's health and well-being is see a doctor of chiropractic. Chiropractic care provides so many things a pregnant body needs: a flexible, balanced spine, hips, and pelvis; good internal organ function without postural stress; and freedom from nerve interference—all essential for a healthy pregnancy and delivery. Along with a better diet, exercise, and avoiding drugs, alcohol, and cigarettes, chiropractic care should be an essential part of a pregnant woman's health care regimen.

A pregnant woman's body needs to be as healthy and strong as possible to handle the rigors of pregnancy and childbirth. Chiropractic care will help ensure that all body systems are functioning properly, especially the reproductive system, which includes the uterus, ovaries, and related organs and structures essential for a healthy pregnancy. If the body's structure is causing the slightest nerve interference to these systems, it could adversely affect the mother and the developing fetus. Your chiropractor will examine your body for distortions also known as subluxations that cause nerve stress and interference. If your chiropractor finds subluxations in your spine and joints, they will correct those distortions with chiropractic adjustments.

In addition, chiropractic care may help with such pregnancy symptoms as nausea and vomiting, allow delivery of full-term infants with ease, and produce overall healthier infants. Chiropractic has demonstrated success with all these issues, as well as back pain and back labor, premature contractions, and malposition of the baby.

WHAT IS THE WEBSTER TECHNIQUE AND HOW DOES IT HELP ME ACHIEVE A MORE BALANCED BODY AND BABY?

The Webster Technique is a specific chiropractic analysis and adjustment that reduces interference to the nervous system and balances maternal pelvic muscles and ligaments. This, in turn, reduces tension in the uterus, increasing space for the baby, and allowing for optimal fetal positioning in preparation for birth. Many pregnant women seek chiropractic care for pregnancy-related neuromusculoskeletal complaints, like lower back pain. The Webster Technique is used most often with pregnant patients because the technique not only assesses for misalignments in the sacral/pelvic region, it also balances the mother's pelvis and soft-tissue structures. This balance may provide a more optimal environment for the baby with positive outcomes for a natural birth.

The current study used a case report of a thirty-year-old nurse-midwife who was thirty-four weeks pregnant with her baby in a transverse (side-to-side) position.

Her previous child was delivered in an occipito-posterior position (the back of the baby's head is against the mother's sacrum). She experienced **major** back labor. The patient came in for chiropractic care because she was experiencing mild, sharp left hip pain and right leg pain.

During her initial exam, the doctor utilized the Webster technique analysis and determined a misalignment in the sacrum and pelvis—he also found misalignments in her neck.

The doctor of chiropractic adjusted the patient's neck with the diversified technique (high-velocity, low-amplitude thrusts); her lower back with the Thompson technique; and her sacrum and pelvis with the modified, diversified technique. Post-check using the Webster analysis showed immediate changes and a balanced sacrum and pelvis.

CAN CHIROPRACTIC CARE LESSEN CHANCES OF INTERVENTION AT BIRTH?

Pregnancy and birth are natural processes, and adding chiropractic care can provide more ease and comfort throughout. There is a long list of benefits to both mother and baby: It prepares the pelvis for an easier pregnancy and birth by creating a state of balance in the pelvis, bony structures, muscles, ligaments and nervous system. It removes torsion or twisting of the ligaments that support the uterus, thus potentially reducing the aberrant tension of the woman's uterus to allow for a more balanced pelvis and easier birth. It reduces the interference to the mother's vital nerve system, which controls and coordinates all her systems and functions, particularly at this special time. It improves the maternal function by decreasing nervous system interference so that her brain can effectively communicate with her body. All of this helps reduce the need for unnecessary interventions at birth. With moms under chiropractic care during the prenatal stages, we see a decrease in labor times and a decrease in interventions.

There are benefits to the infant, as well. It reduces interference to the mother's nerve system to allow for better development of the baby. If the baby is developing in the womb and the mother is in a stressed state, her body chemistry is going to be that of stress. Increased stress hormones flooding through the mother's and baby's circulation will affect the baby's growth and development in utero. This is an important example of how the 3-T's (thoughts) can affect babies early in utero. If the mother is stressed, so is the baby.

Pelvic balance allows greater room for the baby to develop without restrictions to its forming cranium and spine and the other skeletal structures. It also offers the baby room to move into the best possible position for birthing. With proper fetal positioning, there is a significant decrease in dystocia.

Dystocia is a difficult birth, most typically caused by a large or awkwardly positioned baby. This type of birth takes a long time and can make doctors nervous. It is common for doctors to attempt to help this process along by inducing the mother, then during birth, they may feel the need to grasp and pull the head and neck of the baby to get them out, which will cause birth trauma during the delivery process.

Jeanne Ohm DC[xiv] has done extensive studies that show how chiropractic can result in an easier pregnancy, including increased comfort during the third trimester and during the delivery, and a reduced need for analgesics (pain medication). As a result, back labor (contractions and sharp pain felt in the lower back during labor) is significantly less likely. Chiropractic care has helped new mothers become more comfortable breastfeeding (by improving posture), and it has helped them produce more milk. Chiropractic care has also been shown to reduce the likelihood of postpartum depression.

As your pregnancy advances, some chiropractic techniques will need to be modified for your comfort. Your chiropractor is aware of this and will make the necessary changes. In particular, special pregnancy pillows and/or tables with drop-away pelvic pieces are used to accommodate your growing belly. A prenatal chiropractor trained in the proper techniques that address uterine constraint or malpresentations will check for misalignment of the pelvic bones, misalignment of the sacrum and vertebrae, and spasm of the surrounding soft tissues that support the uterus and help hold the pelvis together.

IS CHIROPRACTIC DURING PREGNANCY SAFE?

Absolutely. Many, many pregnant women visit chiropractors during pregnancy each year. Ask around at your local mom groups, birth centers, or birth-preparation classes—or even check out videos online—and you can watch how gentle it is. Not only is it safe, chiropractic has also been proven to lower many risks associated with pregnancy and delivery and comes with many additional benefits for the mother-to-be. Many husbands understand that adding chiropractic care to their pregnant wife's routine keeps them happier, healthier, more relaxed, and feeling great. This is because their nervous system is in an optimal state!

Chiropractic treatment during pregnancy can help mothers manage their changing bodies, which are rapidly shifting out of alignment. Thousands of mothers I know have sworn by chiropractic for relief of back pain and headaches. For others, it has been one of the most effective solutions for combating nausea, while for most it has been essential to ensuring their baby can grow correctly and move into the correct position for delivery.

FIVE REASONS WHY CHIROPRACTIC TREATMENT IS BENEFICIAL DURING PREGNANCY

Keeping the spine and nervous system healthy enables expectant mothers to better handle the stress of childbirth and gives them a greater level of comfort. It is also a drug-free approach to health. Studies show chiropractic care may help decrease labor time by improving functions of the pituitary, adrenal, ovarian, and placental systems. Here's a look at some of the other ways chiropractic care helps expecting mothers:

One: Balance-Added Weight Distribution

As a pregnant mother gains weight, the weight is not evenly distributed. Most of it is added to the front side of her body. Her uterus expands outward during pregnancy, and the center of gravity moves forward, shifting her overall posture. These changes increase pressure on the pelvis and the spine, especially the lumbar and thoracic vertebrae. By improving the functioning of the nervous system, chiropractic treatment empowers the mother's body to respond more effectively to the new weight-distribution paradigm.

Two: Offset the Relaxin Hormone

The hormone relaxin is released during pregnancy to relax ligaments and muscles. Although the resulting malleability creates a softer environment for the growing baby, relaxin also has a downside: it increases the chances that the mother's joints will become misaligned. Chiropractic adjustments offset relaxin release by bringing the mother's joints back into alignment.

Three: Increase Space for Baby

As the fetus grows, ligaments around the pelvis must provide increased support to the uterus. These ligaments often determine how much space the baby has to move in utero. If pelvic ligaments supply symmetrical support, the baby will have more room to move freely, while asymmetrical support from the ligaments limits the available space in the uterus, which can cause the baby to be restricted in their movements, impacting growth, development, and positioning, among other things.

In this sense, chiropractic adjustments reduce the probability that intervention will be required during delivery. During pregnancy, chiropractic treatment improves the alignment of important pelvic ligaments, thereby decreasing the likelihood of diminished space in the pelvis, birth defects, and painful delivery.

Four: Relieve Spinal Subluxation

As stated previously, regardless of whether a woman is pregnant, chiropractic adjustments alleviate or completely rectify spinal subluxation, which happens when the spinal vertebrae move out of position, increasing pressure on nearby spinal nerves. This added pressure causes nerves to malfunction. Why does this matter? Because the nervous system is your body's major communication pathway for messages from the brain. Think about the nervous system as the body's main coordinator. Maximum health comes about when the nervous system can effectively connect with every cell in the body. Subluxation distorts and limits the nervous system's ability to function.

Five: Lower Back Pain Relief

The majority of expectant mothers suffer low back pain, usually due to the shifting biomechanics described earlier. A chiropractor provides spinal manipulations to improve overall spinal alignment, which often brings relief from back pain.

Finally, chiropractic treatment can be conducted safely before and during pregnancy, as well as in the postpartum period. Regular chiropractic adjustments help relieve back pain, enhance nervous system performance, offset prenatal hormones that affect the joints, and prevent diminished space in the womb for the developing baby.

Many people benefit from chiropractic every day, and it's easy to see how the health of both mother and child can be improved and maintained through regular visits to a chiropractor.

AND BEYOND...

INFANTS AND PEDIATRIC CHIROPRACTIC

It has been stated numerous times already, but it's worth stating again, that in childhood, we set the tone for the rest of our lives–physically, chemically, and emotionally. Our formative years prepare us for adulthood in many ways. Pediatric chiropractic encourages proper nervous system function in children, allowing them to meet their developmental milestones and build the foundation of their best health. Yes, healthier children will, in most cases, lead to more robust health in adulthood!

Having your child's nervous system assessed by a pediatric-trained chiropractor as early as possible is one of the best ways to offset any irritation or trauma that occurred during birth. Every birth, no matter how natural or medically invasive, isn't without trauma to the delicate structures of the baby's spine and nervous system. The birth process is straining to both mom and baby. Babies get squeezed out of a small birth canal, sometimes with the assistance of large hands, forceps, or vacuum, or possibly pulled through a small hole in the mother's abdomen. This will cause strain on delicate structures of the upper neck and base of the skull.

Personally, I was blessed to be able to deliver my children's first chiropractic adjustments just moments after their births. In fact, many parents in our practice who know the power of chiropractic make it a priority to have their baby's spine and nervous system checked, often just days after birth.

Our goal is to help children of all ages set the foundation for their amazing life. That means fewer physical problems, emotional disturbances, behavioral issues, better quality sleep, more balanced energy, and healthy timelines for development. We gently and specifically use chiropractic techniques designed to empower children to grow and thrive in their lives. We love helping children of all ages thrive and live happy, healthy lives.

Happy, Healthy Kids

Think of the spine as not just a collection of bones, muscles, and ligaments but an entire neurological "organ" that is the key communication highway between the brain and body. When the brain and body communicate effectively, kids can adapt to their surroundings better. Adaption is the key to a healthy life and why chiropractic care is so helpful to kids. Whether in an infant or someone 100 years old, the inability to adapt to the 3-T's (trauma, toxins, thoughts) is what leads to subluxation.

Optimal health and wellness in children are more than the absence of disease or symptoms. Optimal health is a state of wholeness, and it begins during childhood.

Starting as early as a stressful or straining birth process, children are exposed to a tremendous amount of stress during their first few years. The birthing process is a big and often challenging experience for a delicate baby. Even the most natural birth can create stress patterns in a baby.

Additionally, children encounter countless falls, bumps, and bruises as their bodies grow and try to adapt. Growing takes a lot of work and happens at a very fast pace, especially in the first year. Very commonly, a tight diaphragm muscle or high or low tone of the Vagas nerve can be a culprit in poor digestion in babies and young children. This leads to gas, bloated/distended abdomens, or trouble sleeping. As they grow, their stressors increase. For example, learning to crawl, walk, run, and feel emotions can all be challenging and stressful on their small bodies. When these stressful experiences stack up, their little bodies can develop neurological blockages. As adults, stresses stack up, and children become locked in survival mode (increased Sympathetic Tone or Fight or Flight mode), leading to symptoms, sickness, and disease.

Chiropractic or Medical Doctor?

Both! I applaud Western medicine for life-saving emergency situations; however, when parents ask their MD or pediatrician questions about their child, the answer is often, "They will grow out of it." or "Let's wait and see." This can be less than helpful to parents whose kids are struggling. The bottom line is the pediatrician or medical doctor rarely lays hands on your baby, which is first and foremost in Chiropractic. The word Chiro- means *to do by hands*.

Help Your Child Get Off to a Healthy Start in Life

Our mission is to empower and educate families through high-quality neurological chiropractic care. Through pediatric chiropractic care, we can detect blockages limiting your child's expression of health. Then, we gently correct them, often before symptoms ever show up. Your child is meant to express health, and we can't wait to help them thrive naturally!

I advocate that EVERY child gets checked by a pediatric chiropractor whether they have symptoms or not. Getting your kids checked regularly by a pediatric chiropractor can ensure your child's body is moving and functioning well.

If your kiddo has headaches, irritable bowel syndrome, constipation, delayed or irregular crawling patterns, flat sides of their head, re-occurring ear infections, emotional outbursts, or sensitivity to foods, clothes, or environment, please find a pediatric chiropractor to have them checked.

If your kiddo is perfect, eats well, sleeps well, and meets all their developmental milestones, please check them. The spine and nervous system are the window to how well our babies are adapting in life, and adaption is the measure of true health. Chiropractic is all about HEALTH, and the best support for the body at any age is through chiropractic care.

REASONS FOR YOUR CHILD TO BE CHECKED BY A CHIROPRACTOR

BABIES	TODDLERS
- Nursing Issues - Reflux and excessive spitting up - Stiffness and Tightness - Colic - Gas pains and constipation - Torticollis and abnormal head shape - Milestones and growth - Wellness	- Ear Infections - Congestions, cough and excessive colds - Sleep issues - Eczema - Speech development - Coordination and balance
KIDS	TEENS
- ADHA - Anxiety - Asthma - Sensory Processing - Growing Pains - Bed Wetting - Sleep - Behavior & Emotions	- Headaches - Anxiety - Depression - Sleep - Hormones - Sports Performance - Academic Performance - Focus - Mood

NEXT STEPS

I hope you have found valuable information, had questions answered, thought of new questions, and discovered methods to help you wherever you are in your process, from preconception to pregnancy to life-long health.

This book has presented the Trauma (structural or physical trauma), Toxins (chemicals), and Thoughts (mental/emotional) components of preconception, pregnancy, and beyond and shows how each is related to the other, connecting us to true health. If any one of these components is not in a healthy state, it will affect the entire status of the mother and growing baby. Likewise, the father plays a crucial role in this process, because it does take both mother and father to create life.

After being in private practice for over fifteen years and witnessing how the parents' health impacts their children, I am on a mission to bring awareness to this important piece of the puzzle that is not often talked about. Our children are our future! Starting them with the best health possible will give them an edge in life, influencing the entire planet and future generations.

For more resources and to get started with taking steps towards your newfound health journey for you and your family, I invite you to visit
http://www.keoughchiropractic.com/

BIOGRAPHY

Dr. Felicity Keough-Bligh is a mother, wife, and holistic family physician proficient in manual medicine and chiropractic, and a passionate advocate for improving the health of women and children. She is an author, speaker, and owner of a successful prenatal, pediatric, and family wellness clinic in the Midwest. Dedicated to lifelong wellness, her mission is to serve, teach, and inspire her patients so they can attain their full potential and sustain optimal health.

http://www.keoughchiropractic.com/

I'd love it if you could please leave a review of my book via this QR code!

ENDNOTES

i. What is Epigenetics? | CDC

ii. The Microbiome | The Nutrition Source | Harvard T.H. Chan School of Public Health

iii. National Survey of Children's Health (NSCH) 2018 19:Number of Current or Lifelong Health Conditions, Nationwide, Age in Three Groups website. childhealthdata.org (Accessed February 24, 2021)

iv. MTHFR Gene, Folic Acid, and Preventing Neural Tube Defects | CDC

v. The Institute for Functional Medicine | Information and educational seminars and conferences on functional medicine. (ifm.org)

vi. Health and Economic Costs of Chronic Diseases | CDC

vii. Allopathic medicine is the general term for what most people understand as modern, Western medicine. The allopathic medicine definition describes it as a method of treating disease with remedies (such as surgery or drugs) that produce different effects from those caused by the disease.

viii. https://www.ifm.org/functional-medicine/what-is-functional-medicine/

ix. Reprinted with permission by Felicity Keough-Bligh from Healing From Within p.8

x. Colburg, Sheri R. "How to Increase Insulin Sensitivity." December 2008. (Accessed September 2019) https://www.diabetesselfmanagement.com/managing-diabetes/treatment-approaches/increasing-insulin-sensitivity/

xi. Godman, Heidi. "Regular exercise changes the brain to improve memory, thinking skills." April 2014. (Accessed September 2019) https://www.health.harvard.edu/blog/regular-exercise-changes-brain-improve-memory-thinking-skills-201404097110

xii. https://www.manhattangastroenterology.com/exercise-affects-digestion/ (Accessed September 2019)

xiii. https://www.wonderopolis.org/wonder/how-many-breaths-do-you-take-each-day (Accessed September 2019)

xiv. Lowenstein, Jason E. "How to Correct Anterior Pelvic Tilt (& Lumbar Lordosis)." (Accessed September 2024) https://jasonlowensteinmd.com/how-to-correct-anterior-pelvic-tilt-lumbar-lordosis/

xv. https://pathwaysoffamilywellness.org/item/jeanne-ohm-dc.html

www.ingramcontent.com/pod-product-compliance
Lightning Source LLC
Chambersburg PA
CBHW071723020426
42333CB00017B/2372